INSIDE MY BODY
LUNGS

WRITTEN BY JODY JENSEN SHAFFER ILLUSTRATED BY TERESA ALBERINI

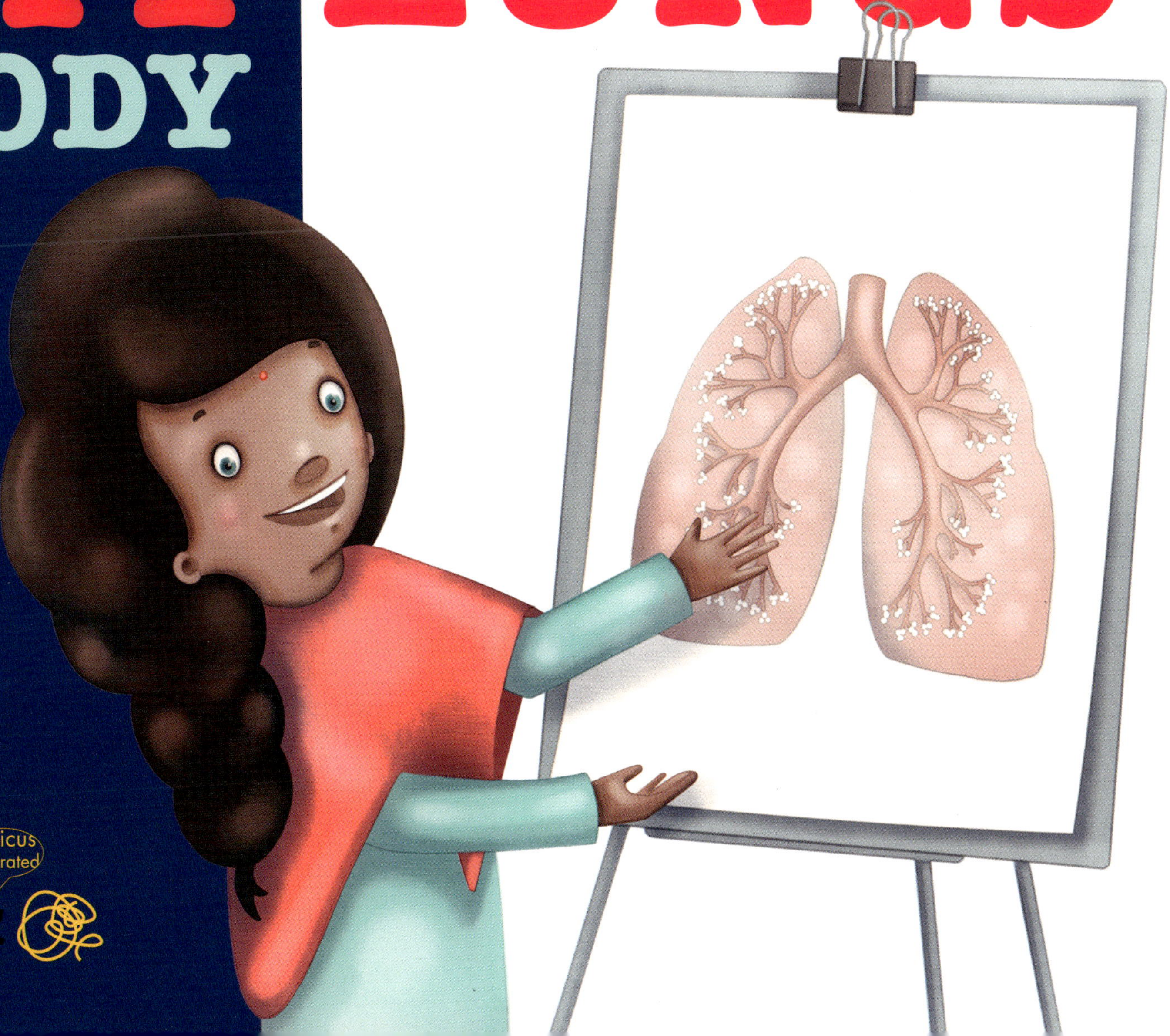

amicus illustrated

amicus illustrated

Amicus Illustrated is published by Amicus
P.O. Box 1329, Mankato, MN 56002
www.amicuspublishing.us

Library of Congress Cataloging-in-Publication Data
Shaffer, Jody Jensen, author.
My lungs / by Jody Jensen Shaffer ; illustrated by Teresa Alberini.
pages cm. -- (Inside my body) (Amicus illustrated)
Summary: "A girl named Jasmine teaches a younger student at her school everything she has learned about lungs and the respiratory system while researching them for her booth at her school's science fair"-- Provided by publisher.
Audience: K to grade 3.
ISBN 978-1-60753-756-4 (library binding) -- ISBN 978-1-60753-855-4 (ebook)
1. Lungs--Juvenile literature. 2. Human physiology--Juvenile literature. [1. Respiratory system.] I. Alberini, Teresa, illustrator. II. Title.
QP121.S53 2016
612.2'4--dc23 2014041503

Editor: Rebecca Glaser
Designer: Kathleen Petelinsek

Printed in the United States of America at Corporate Graphics in North Mankato, Minnesota.

10 9 8 7 6 5 4 3 2 1

ABOUT THE AUTHOR

Jody Jensen Shaffer is the author of 19 books of fiction and nonfiction for children. She also writes poetry, stories, and articles for children's magazines. When she is not writing, Jody copy edits and proofreads for children's publishers. She tries to keep her body healthy by walking regularly and eating nutritious foods. Visit Jody on the web at jodyjensenshaffer.blogspot.com.

ABOUT THE ILLUSTRATOR

Teresa Alberini has always loved painting and drawing. She attended the Academy of Fine Arts in Florence, Italy, and she now lives and works as an illustrator in a small town on the Italian coast. Visit her on the web at www.teresaalberini.com.

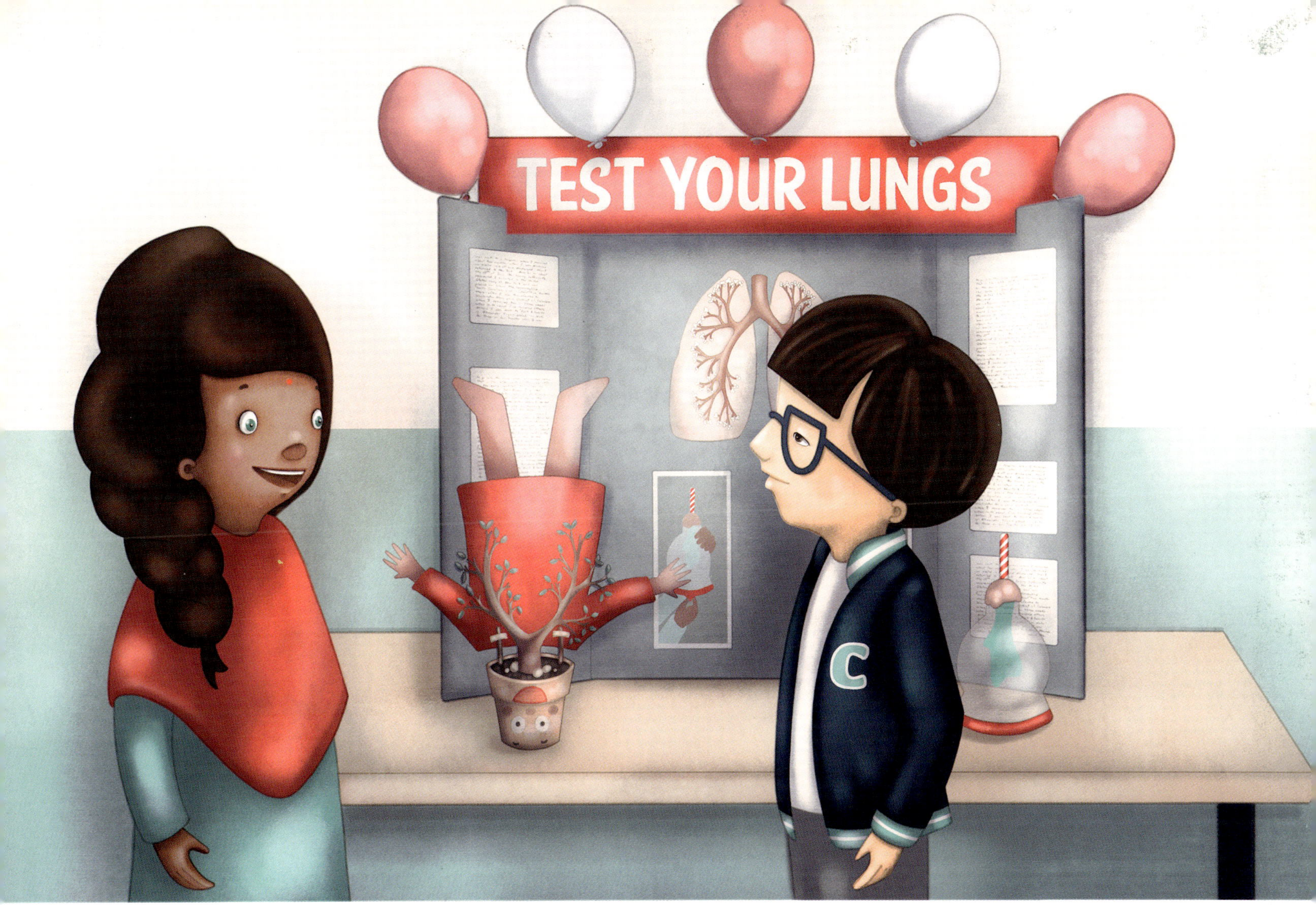

"Nice science fair project, Jasmine!"

"Thanks. Do you want blow up a balloon to test your lungs, Jet?"

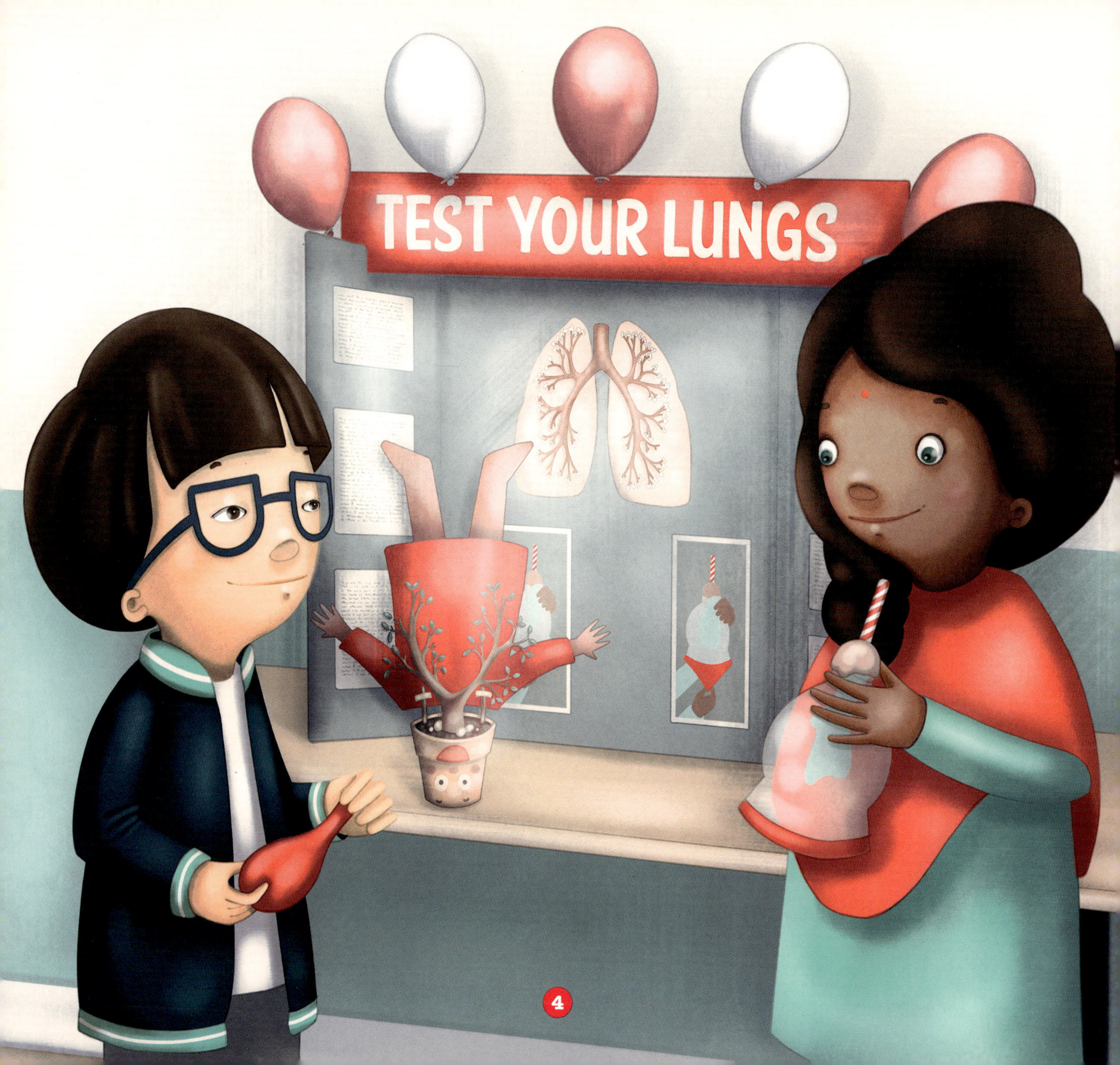
TEST YOUR LUNGS

"But I breathe through my nose and mouth. How does blowing up a balloon test my lungs?"

"The air goes from your mouth and nose into your windpipe. It's like this straw."

"And then the air goes into my lungs?"

"Yes. But that's not the whole story, Jet."

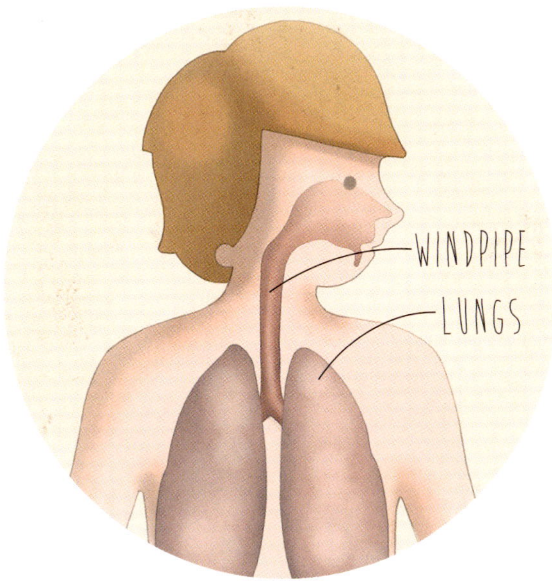

"Your diaphragm muscle helps too. It's like this bottom balloon in my model. The diaphragm moves down and then your lungs can take in air."

"And then I breathe out."

"Yes. But first, the air travels through your body."

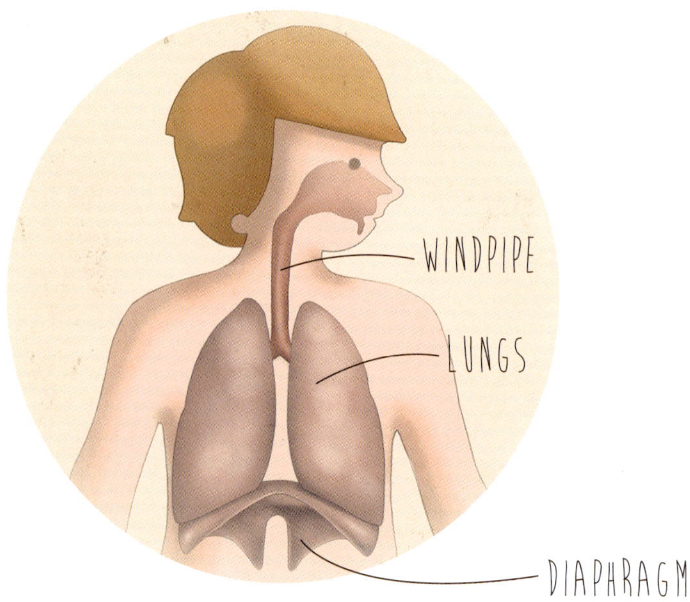

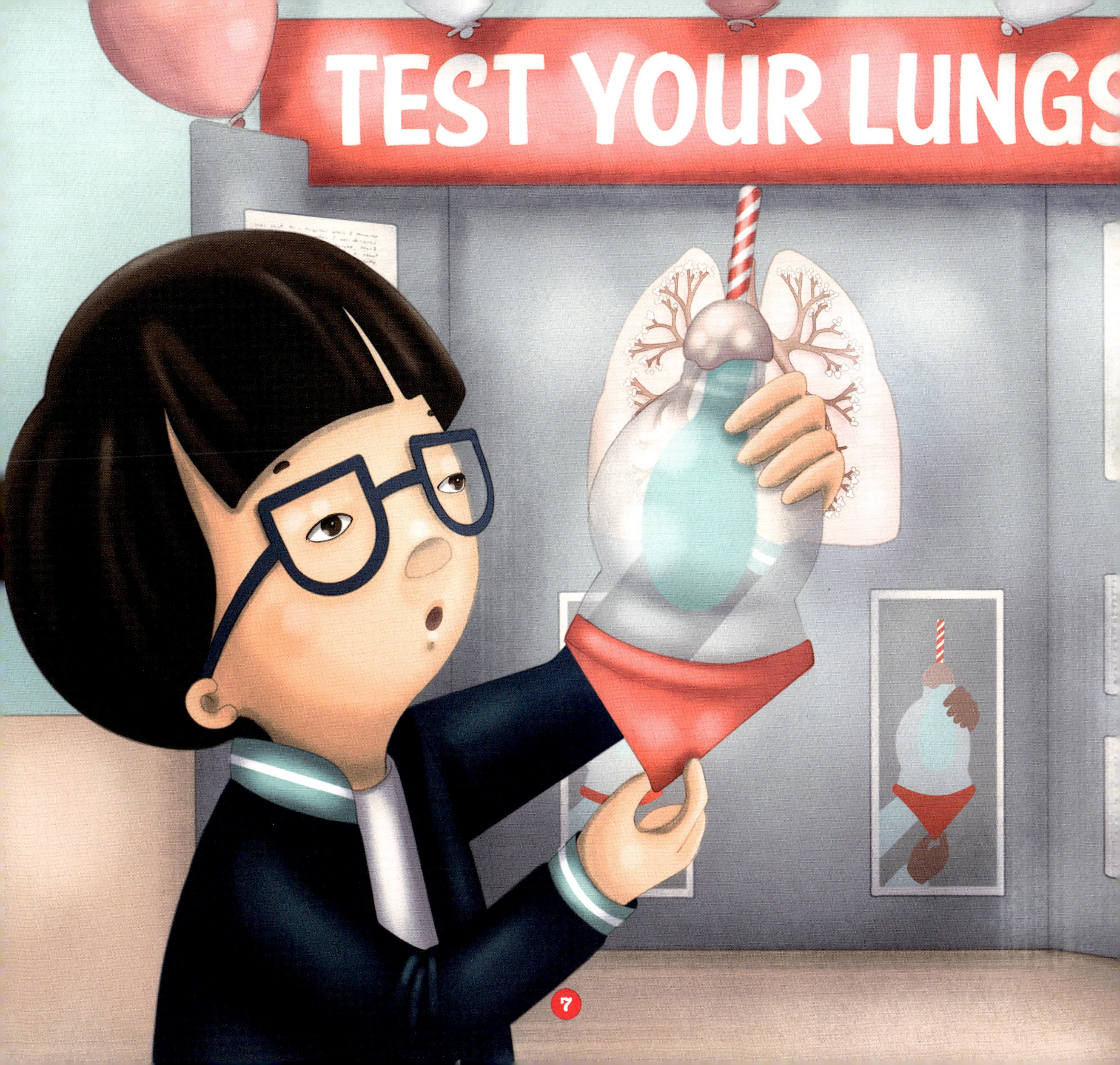
TEST YOUR LUNGS

"In your lungs, the air splits from the windpipe at the bronchi and travels through the bronchioles. The tubes get smaller and smaller."

"Like the branches on your little tree."

"Exactly!"

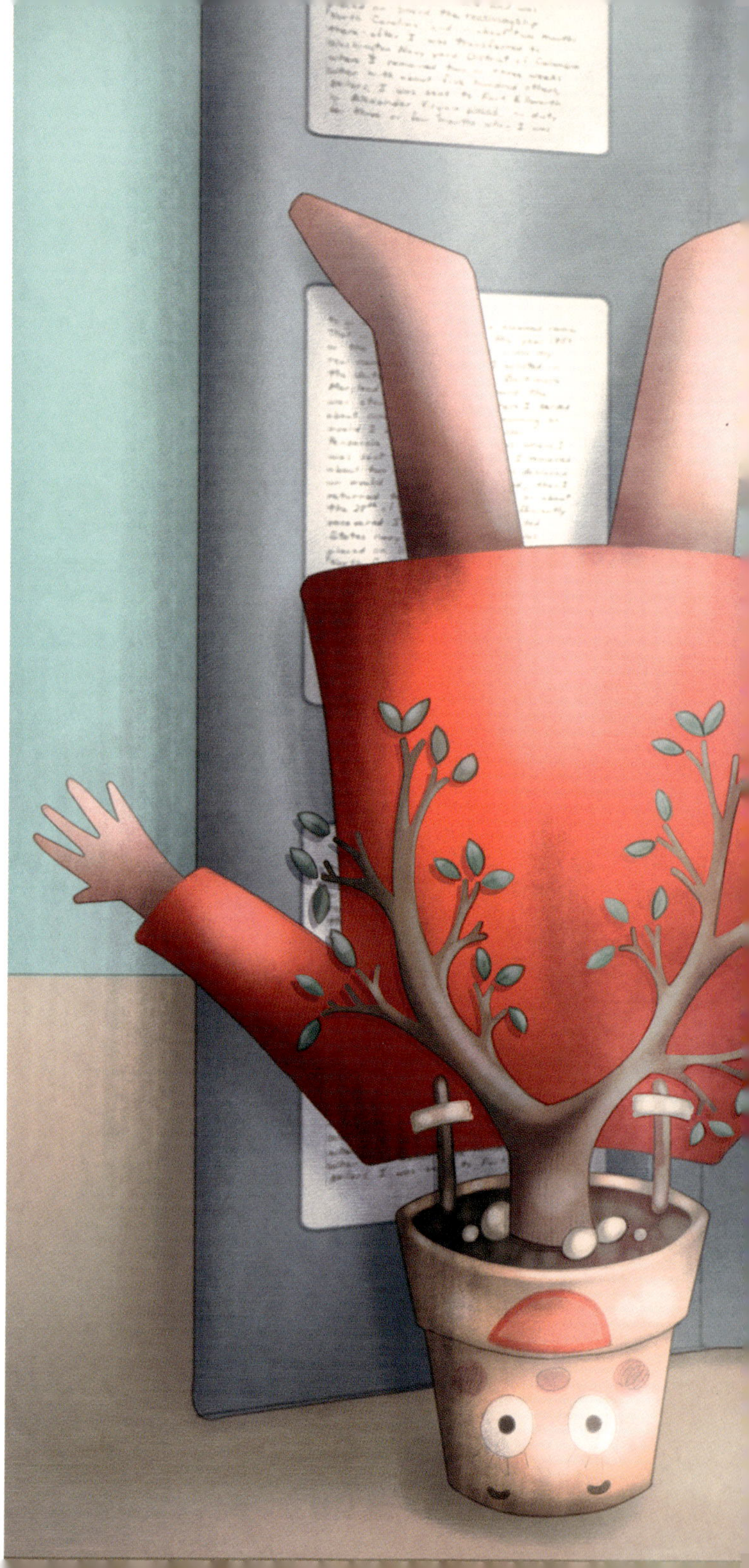

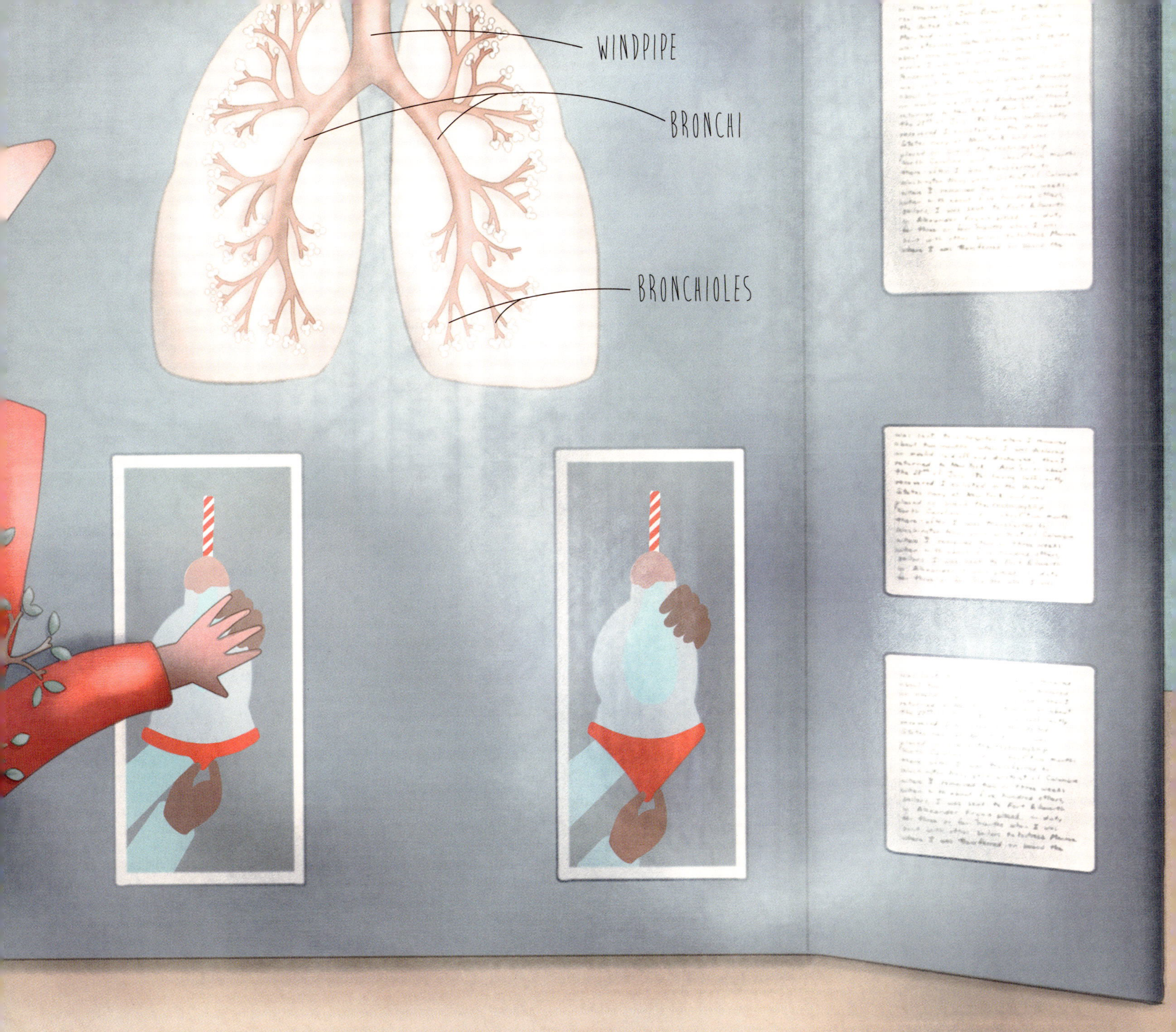
WINDPIPE
BRONCHI
BRONCHIOLES

"Then what happens?"

"The tubes end at tiny air sacs called alveoli."

"They look like tiny grapes."

"Yes, but they give oxygen to your blood. Then your blood takes it to the rest of your body."

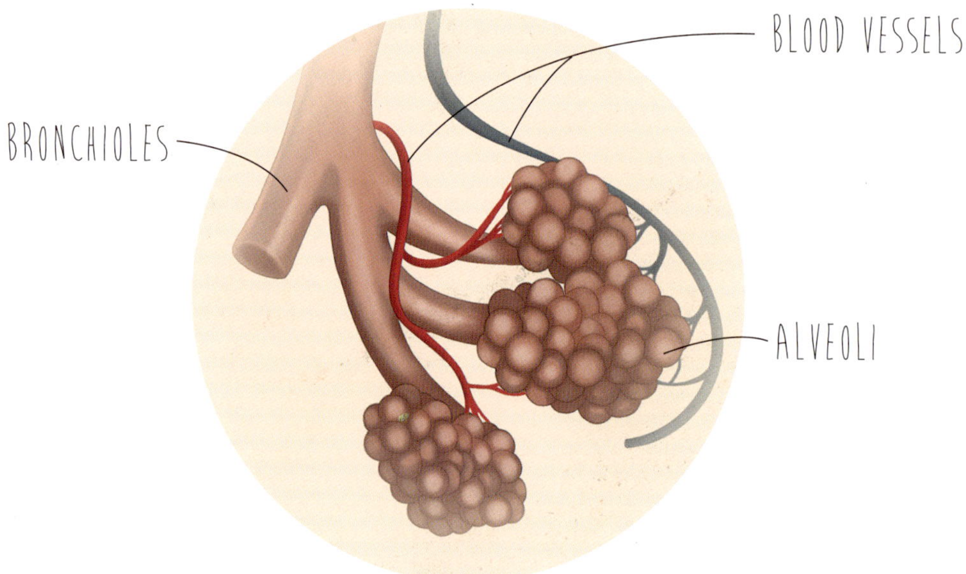

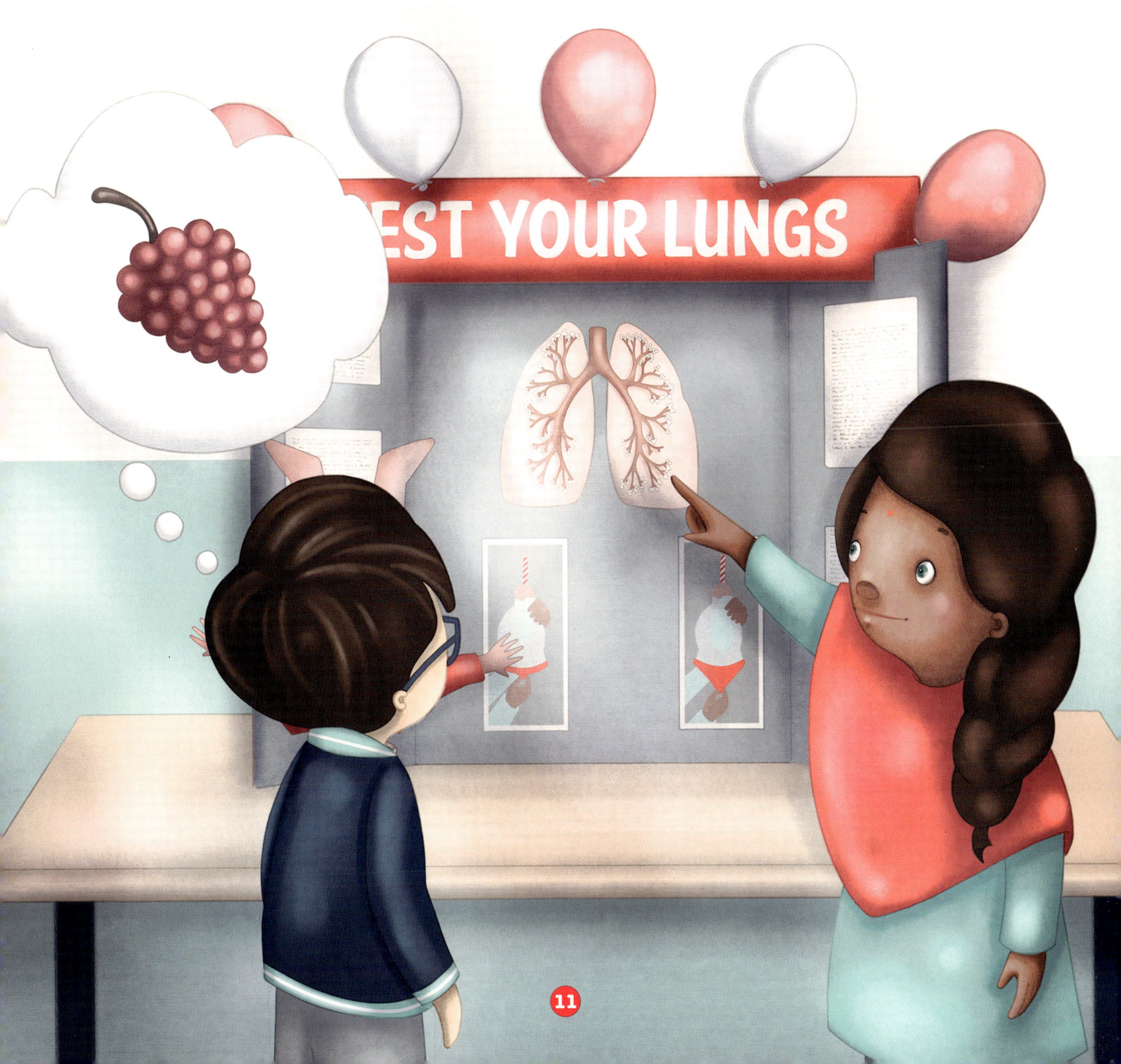
EST YOUR LUNGS

"What about breathing out?"

"After your body uses up the oxygen, the blood is left with carbon dioxide. Your body needs to get rid of that."

"So your body trades carbon dioxide for oxygen?"

"That's right."

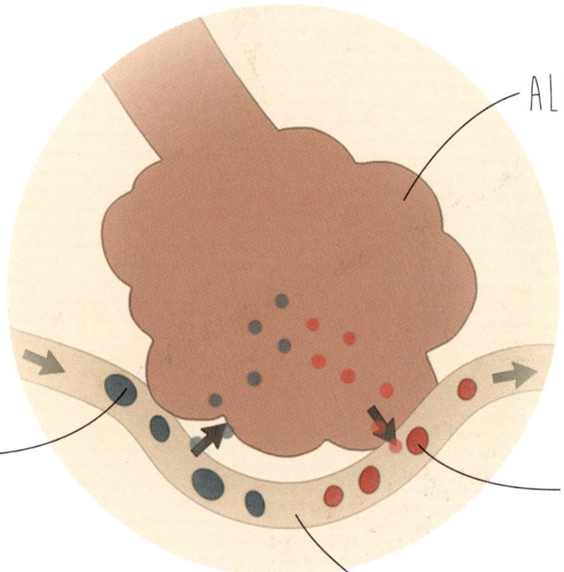

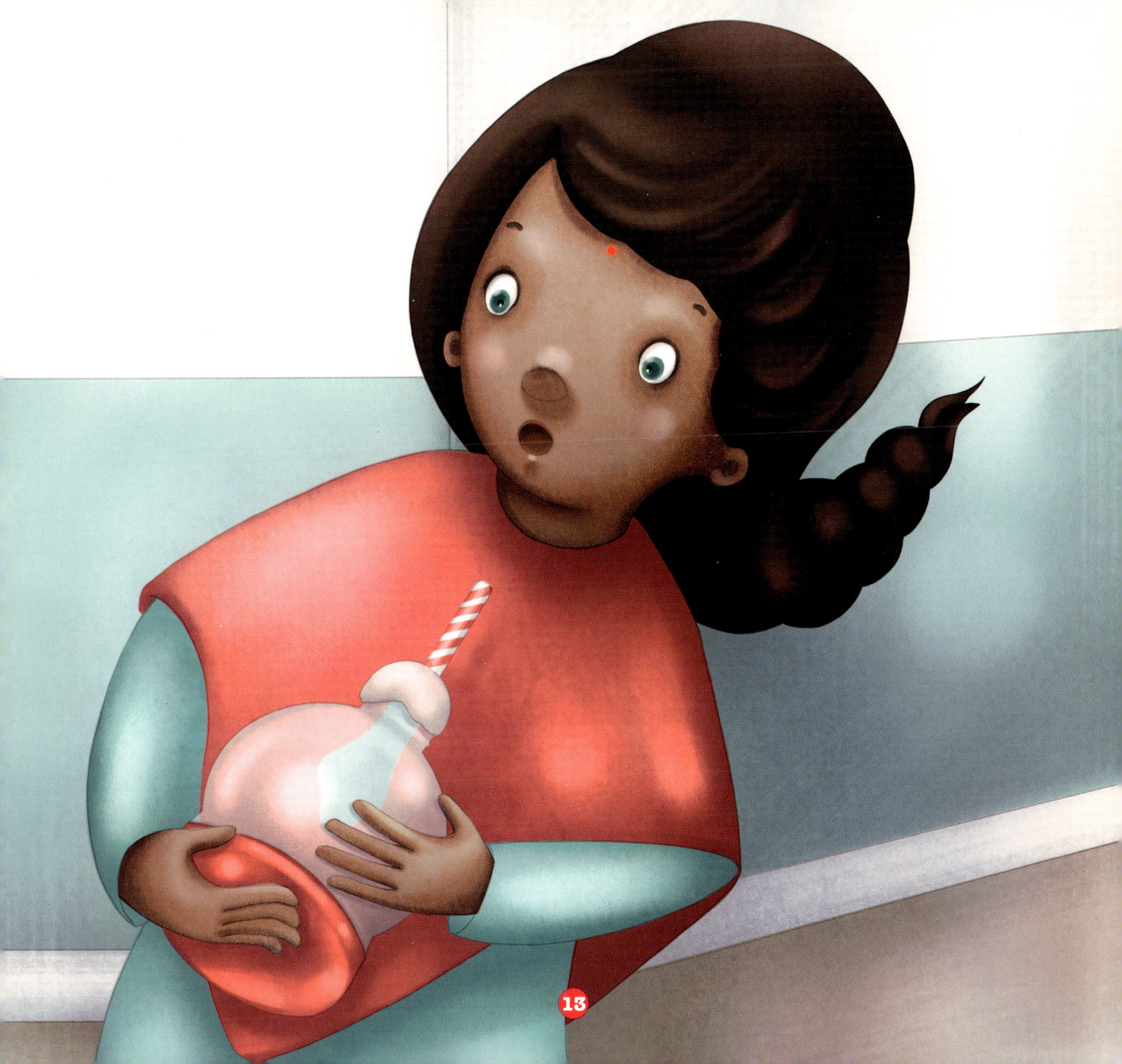

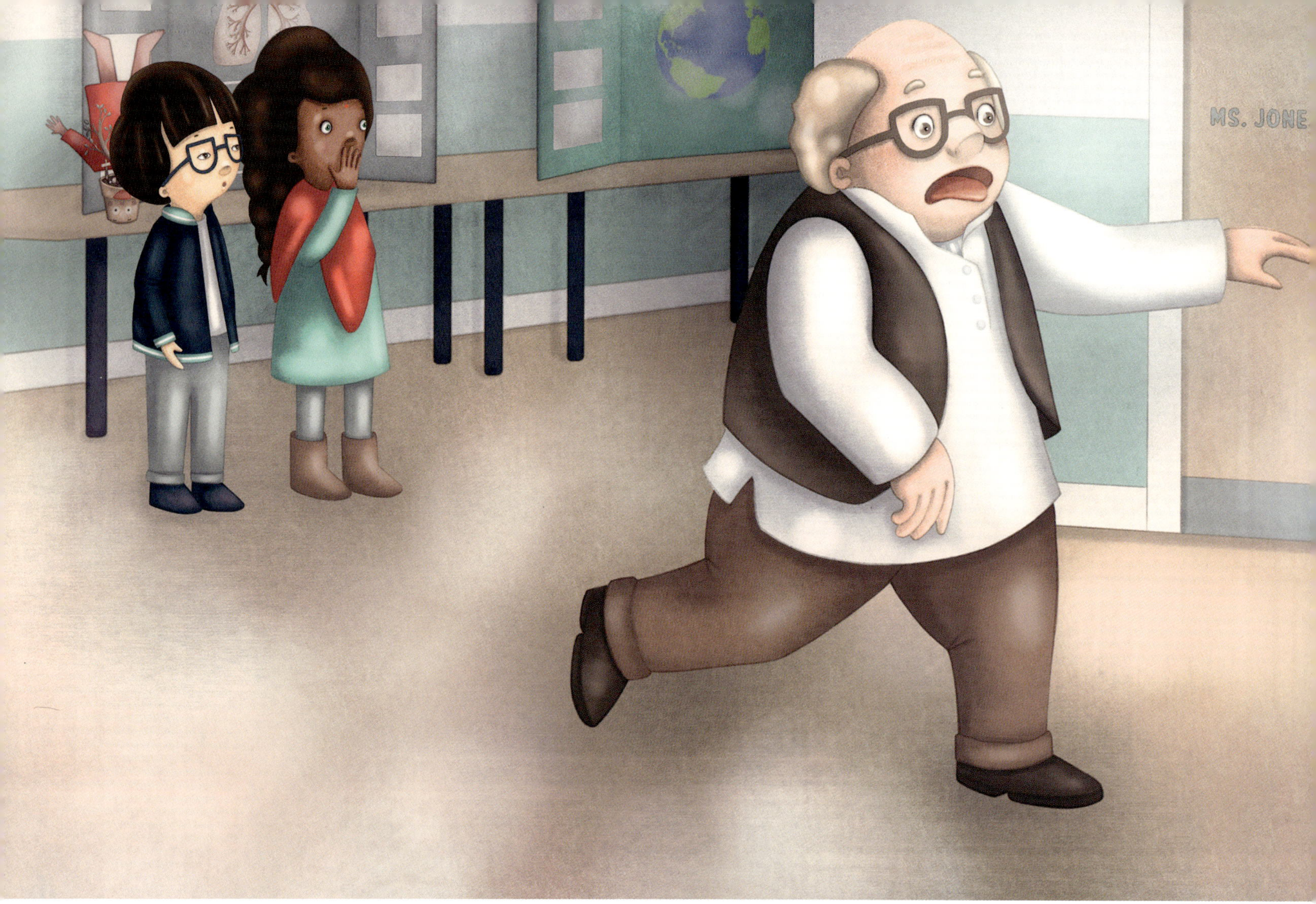

“Why does my body need oxygen?”

“Your muscles need oxygen to move. Look at Mr. Brown! His lungs are working really hard.”

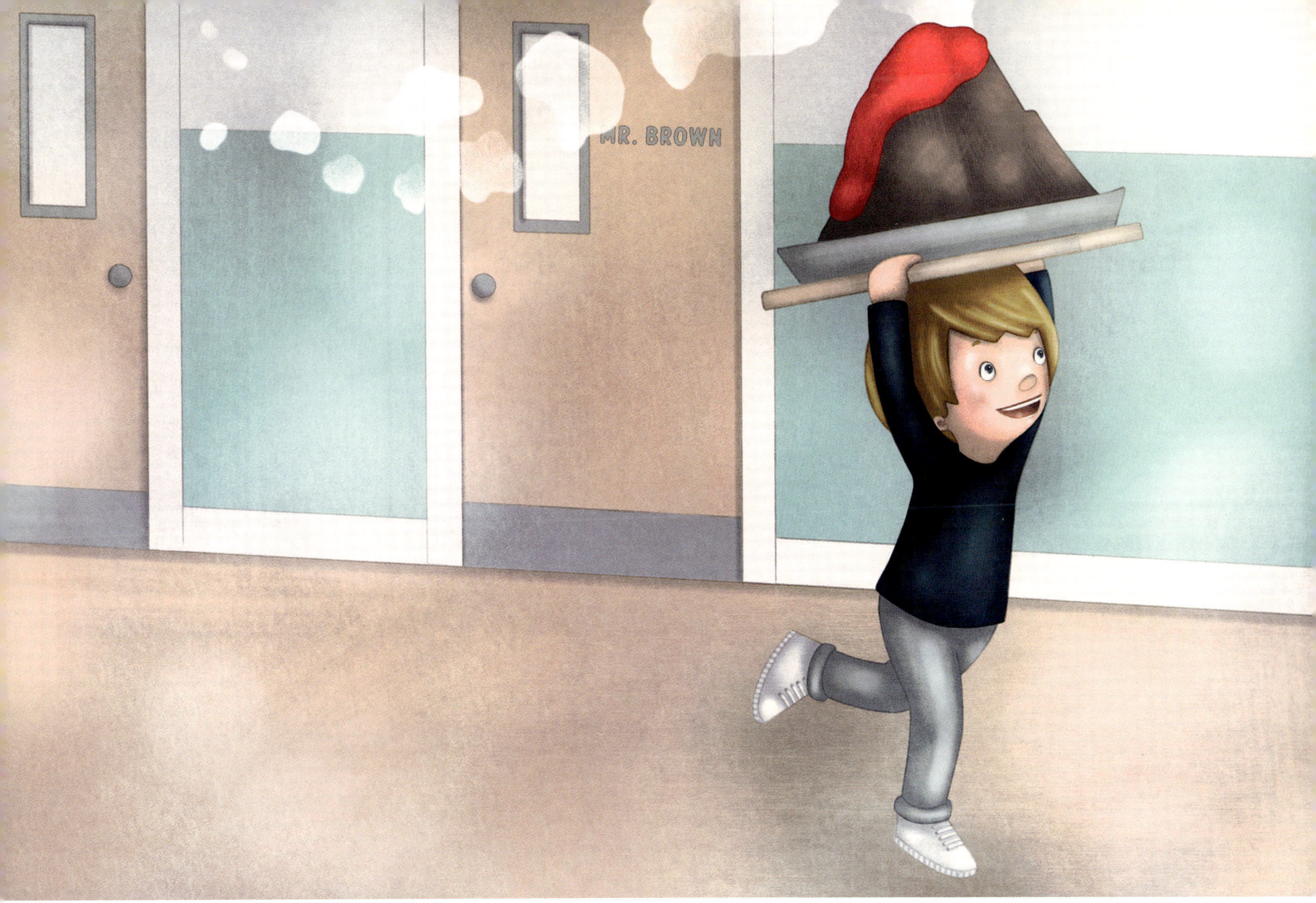

"That's how I feel after soccer practice!"

"The more you exercise, the healthier your lungs will be."

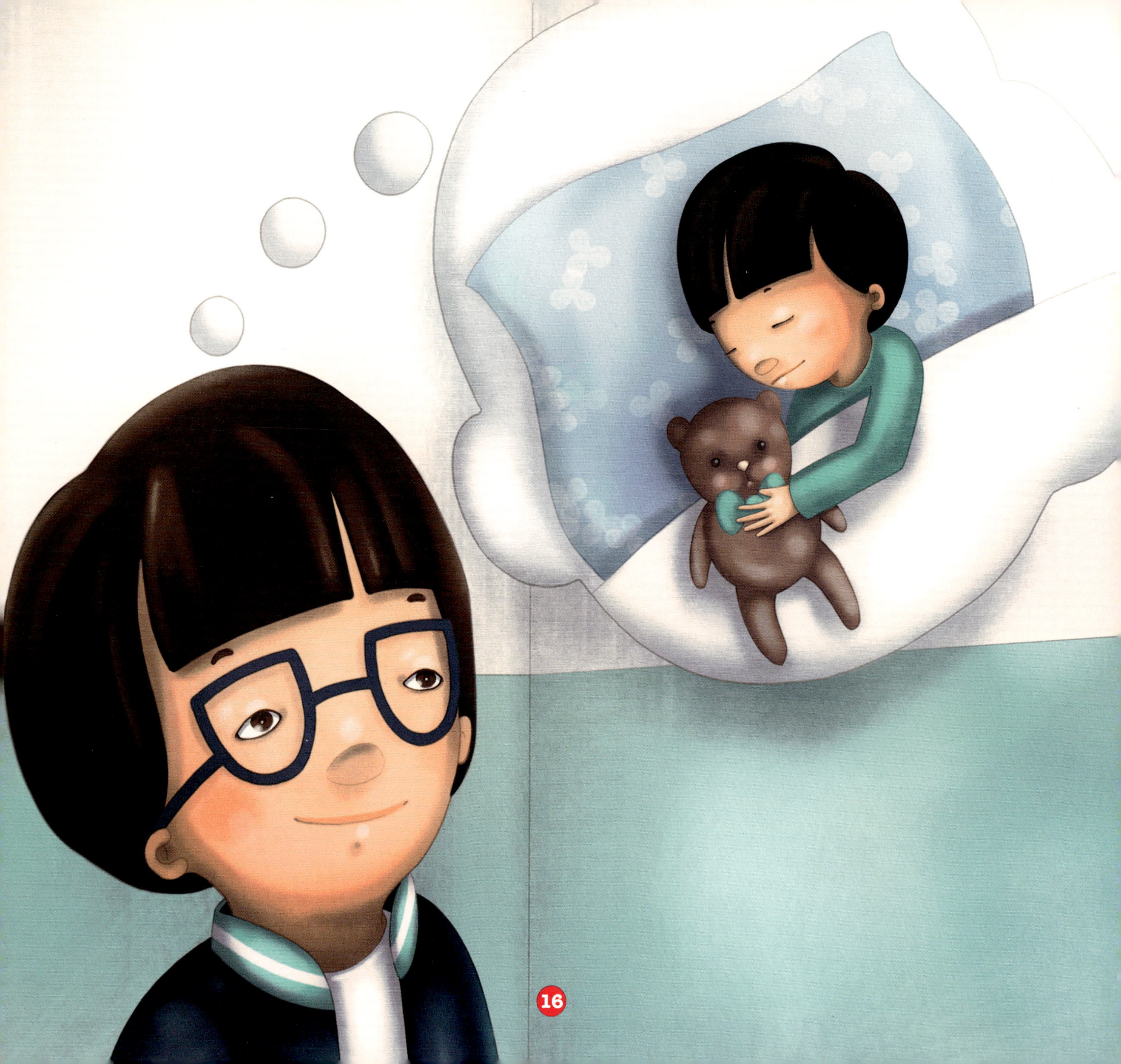

“What about when I’m *not* exercising?”

“Your muscles, organs, and brain need oxygen all the time, Jet.”

“Even when I’m sleeping?”

“Yes. You don’t have to think about breathing. Your brain tells your lungs how much oxygen it needs.”

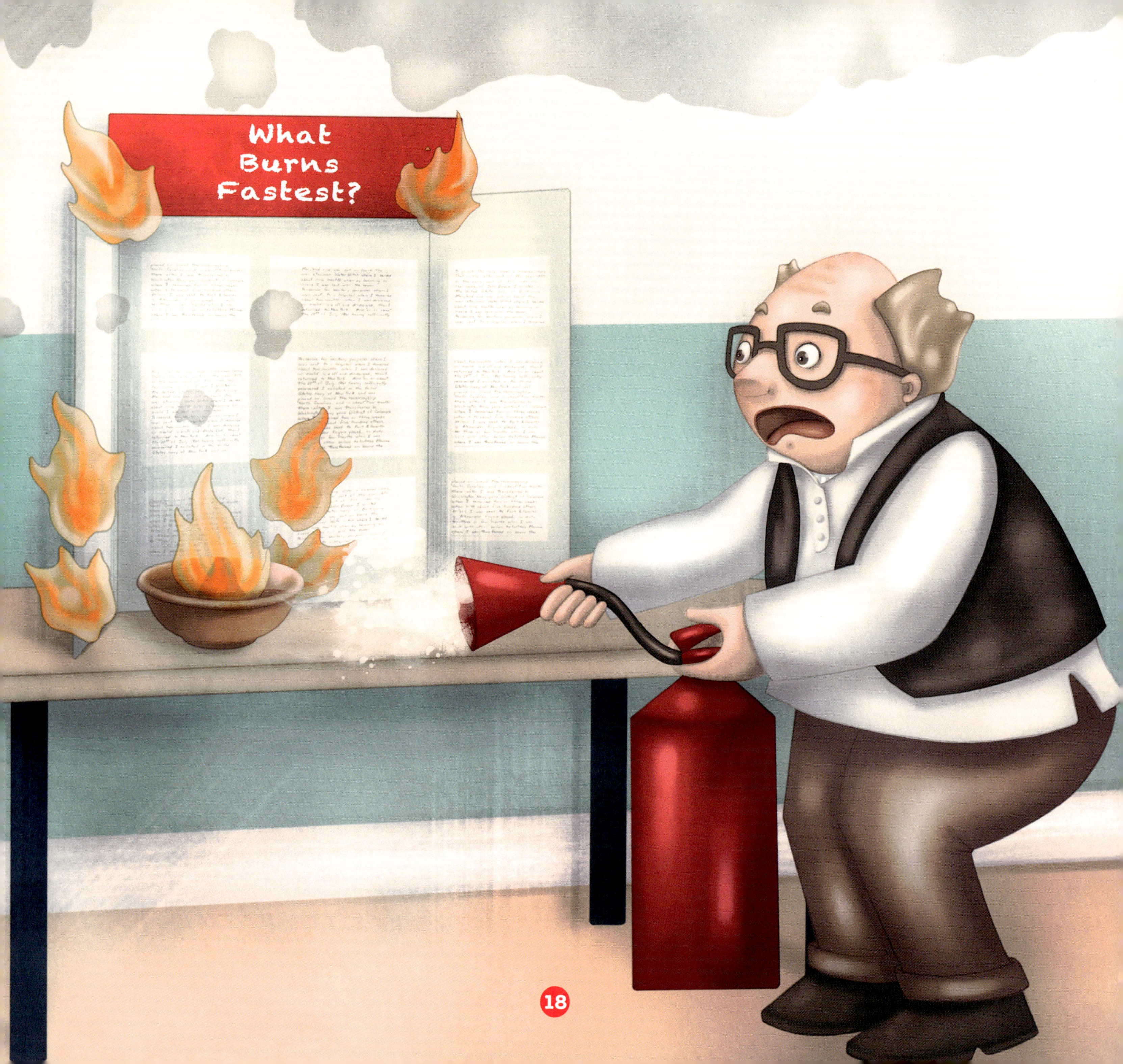
What Burns Fastest?

"Oh no! David's project is on fire! Don't breathe the smoke. It will irritate your lungs."

"It's making me cough."

"Coughing will help. Small hairs in your lungs, the cilia, clear out the smoke. But too much irritation can damage the hairs."

"Thanks for teaching me about the lungs, Jasmine!"

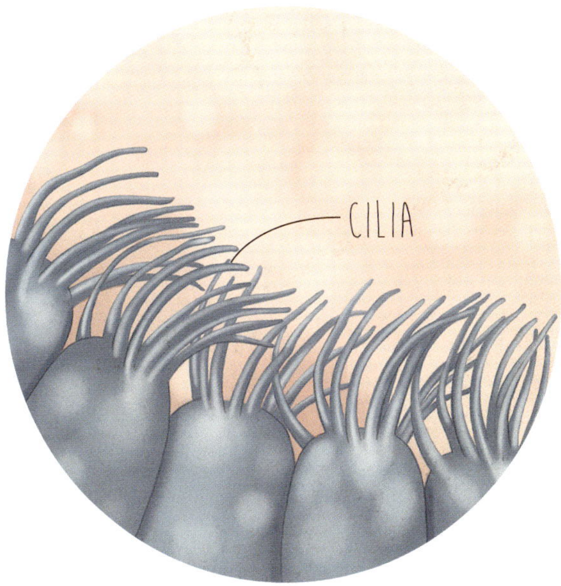

"But wait! Did you know the diaphragm can jerk and make your lungs take in quick gasps of air? That's what causes hiccups. You can try to stop them by holding your breath or getting a sudden . . ."

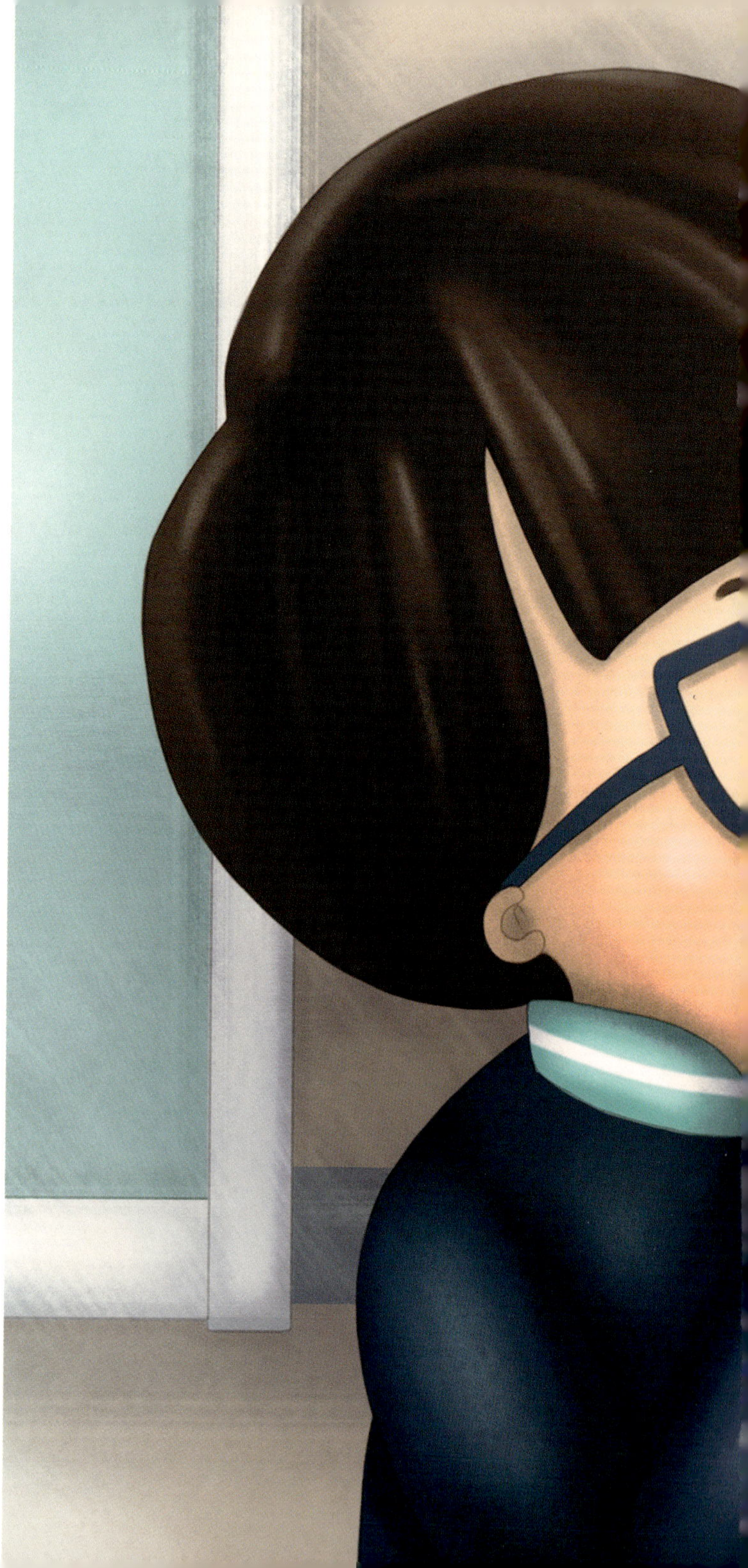

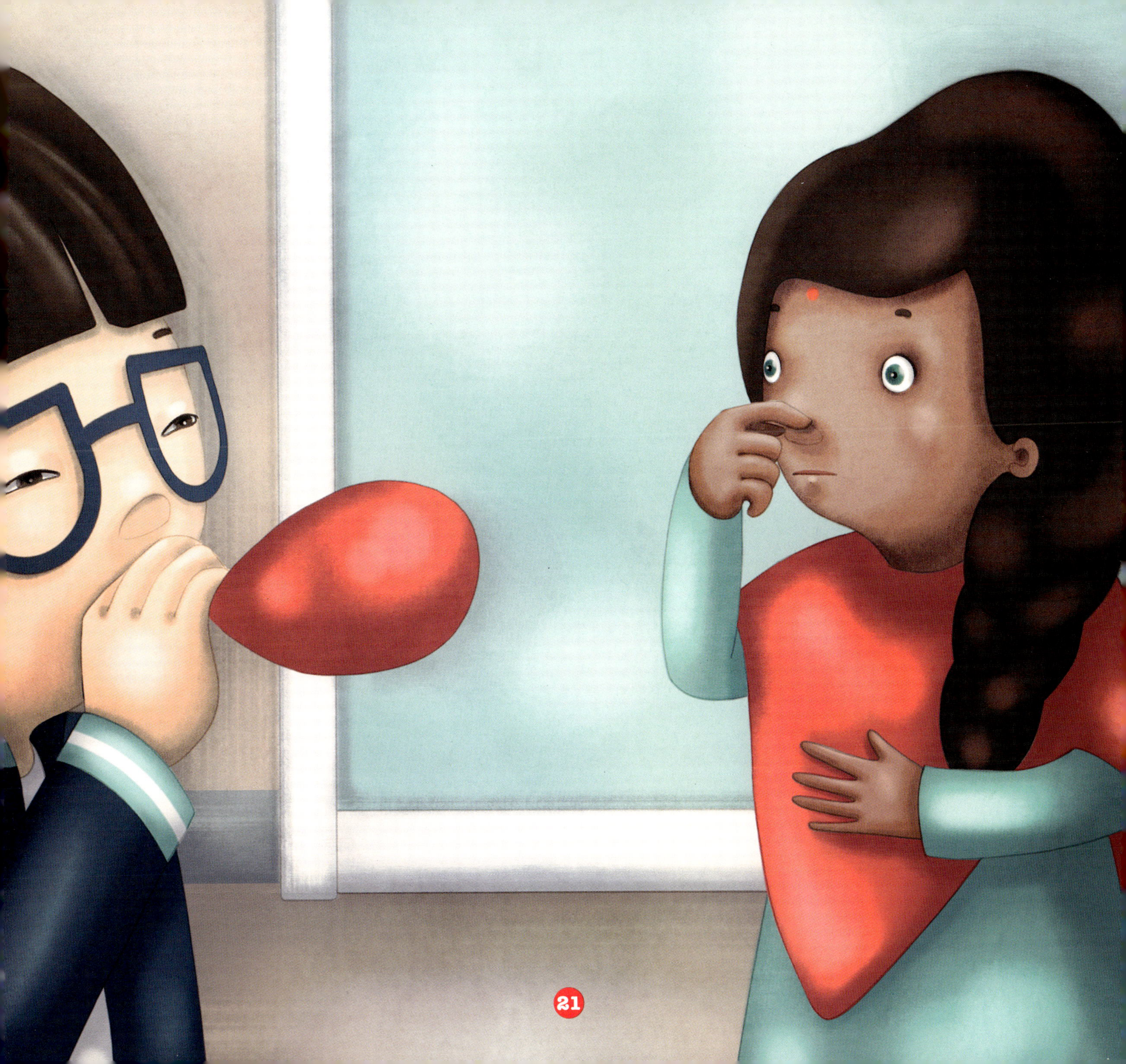

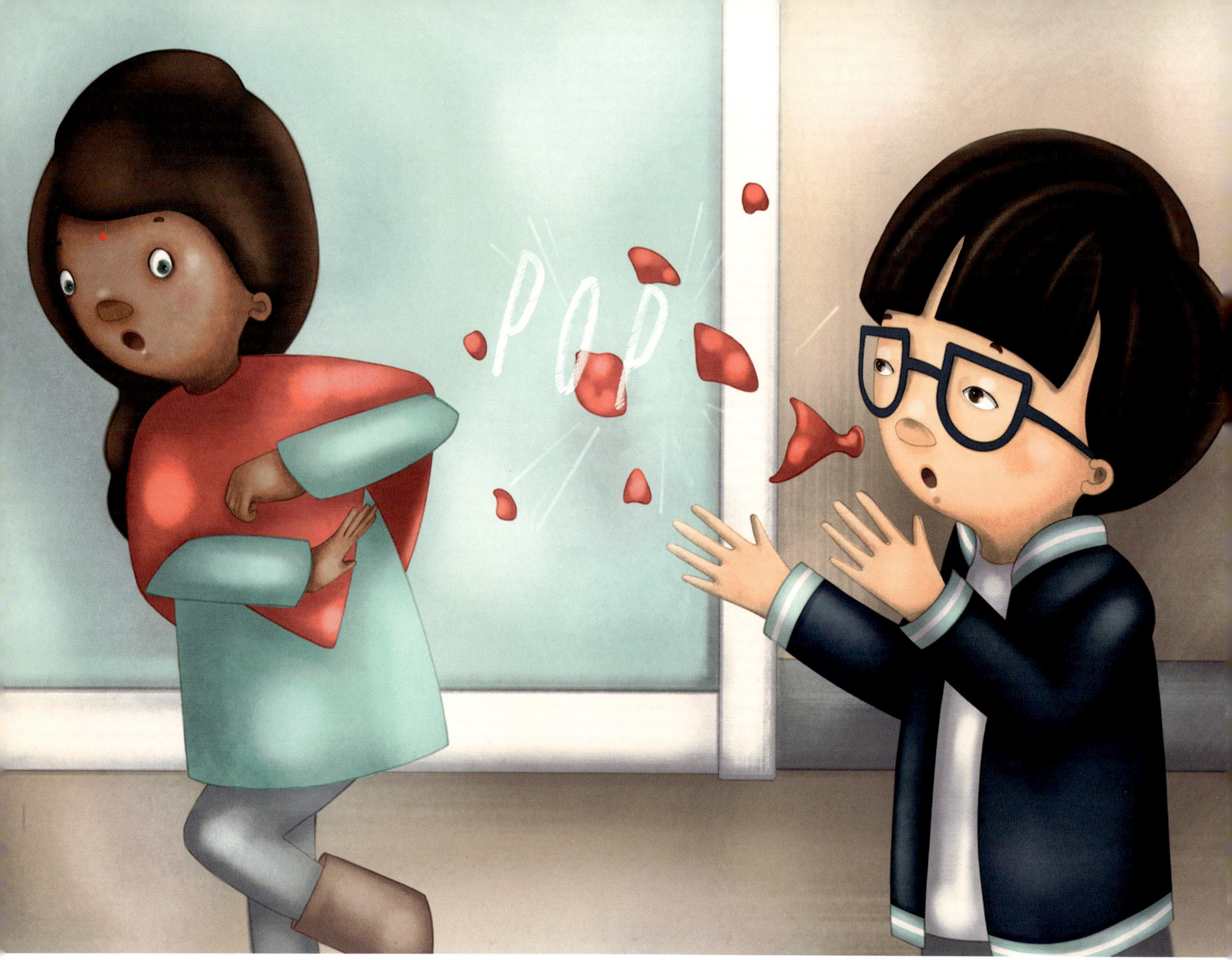

"... surprise!"

BODY BY THE NUMBERS

Alveoli - 600 million

Bronchi - 2

Bronchioles - 30,000 in each lung

Diaphragm - 1

Lungs - 2

Mouth - 1

Nose - 1

Windpipe - 1

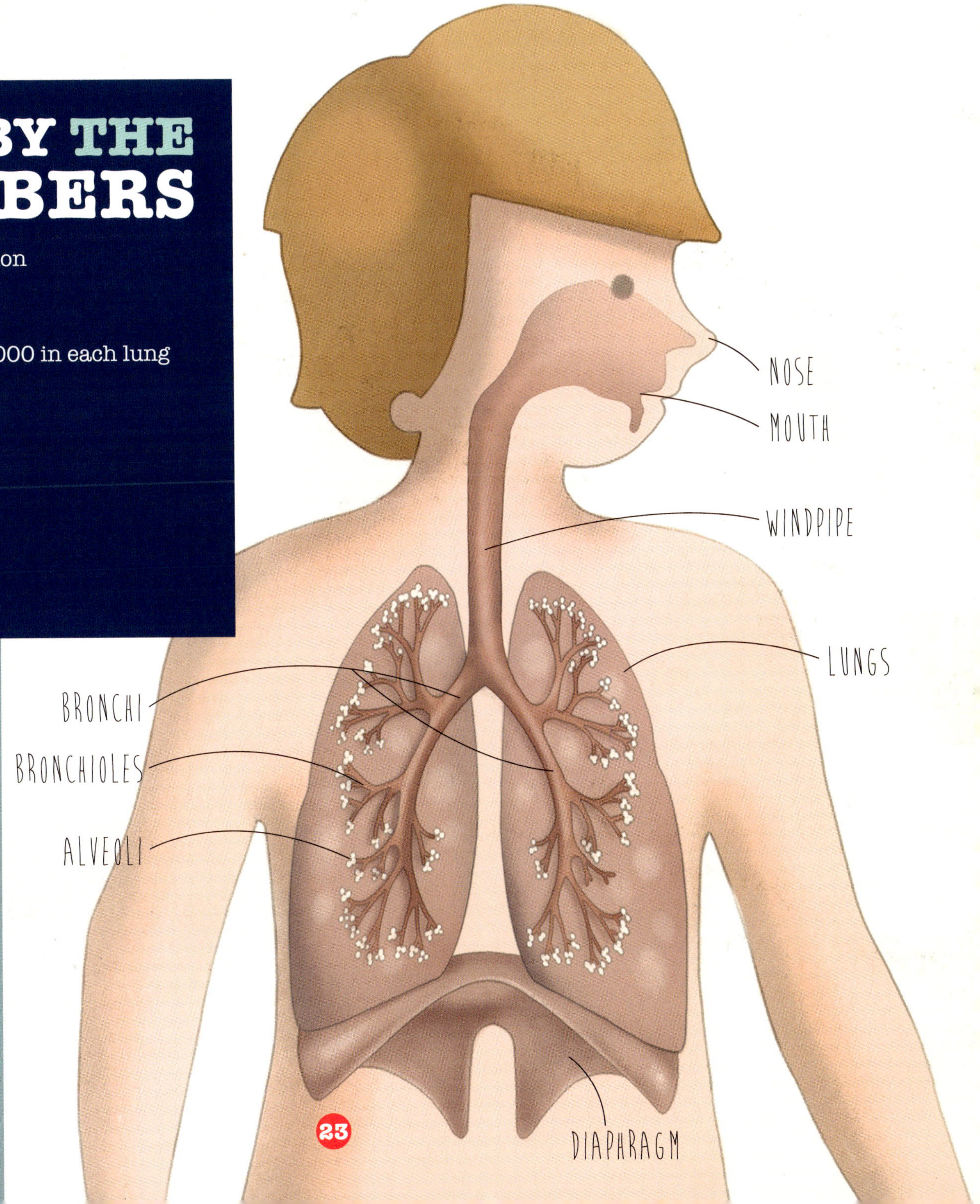

GLOSSARY

alveoli—Tiny air sacs in the lungs where the exchange of oxygen and carbon dioxide takes place.

bronchi—Two air tubes that connect the windpipe to the lungs.

bronchioles—Tiny tubes that branch out into the lungs and carry oxygen.

lungs—Two organs within the ribcage that receive and use oxygen.

READ MORE

Brett, Flora. **Your Respiratory System Works!** North Mankato, Minn.: Capstone Press, 2015.

Figorito, Christine. **The Lungs in Your Body**. New York: Britannica Educational Publishing, 2015.

Gardner, Jane P. **Take a Closer Look at Your Lungs**. Mankato, Minn.: Child's World, 2013.

Halvorson, Karin. **Inside the Lungs**. Minneapolis: ABDO Pub., 2013.

WEBSITES

Inside Our Bodies: How Our Lungs Work
www.howourlungswork.com/index.html
Explore all the different parts of your lungs and find out what they do.

KidsHealth: Your Lungs & Respiratory System
kidshealth.org/kid/htbw/lungs.html
Read more information about your lungs and breathing.

Science Sparks: Fake Lung Experiment
www.science-sparks.com/2012/04/13/breathing-making-a-fake-lung/
Build a lung model like Jasmine's to see how the lungs work.